Contents

Purpose of this document 1

What is clinical research? 2

Why do people choose to participate in research? 3

What are the different types of clinical research? 5

What are the risks and benefits of participating in research? 8

What rights do I have? 11

What are the possible financial costs? 12

Who can participate in clinical research? 12

What is randomization? 13

What is informed consent? 14

What else should I consider? 15

How do researchers make sure that participants are safe? 16

What kinds of results will come from the research? 18

How can I enroll in clinical research? 19

What kinds of questions should I ask the researcher? 20

Glossary 21

References 24

For more information on clinical research and clinical trials 25

Purpose of this document

Choosing to take part in clinical research is an important personal decision. Your decision to participate will depend on your interests, needs, and expectations about research.

This brochure, prepared by the National Institute of Mental Health (NIMH), provides answers to common questions about volunteering for mental health clinical research. NIMH is part of the National Institutes of Health (NIH), the primary Federal agency for conducting and supporting medical research.

Our goal is to give you basic information about clinical research and help you make a decision about whether to participate. Please review this information and discuss it with those close to you. As you read, write down questions you may want to ask.

How to use this guide:

This document provides an overview about participating in clinical research. To get details on a study, it is important to bring any questions and concerns to the researchers who are doing the study. For example, only the researchers can answer questions about whether a participant will be able to stay on medications or will be compensated for taking part in the study. You may wish to review the glossary first to become familiar with some of the terms used in clinical research studies.

A glossary is included at the end of this document. As you read, write down questions you may want to ask.

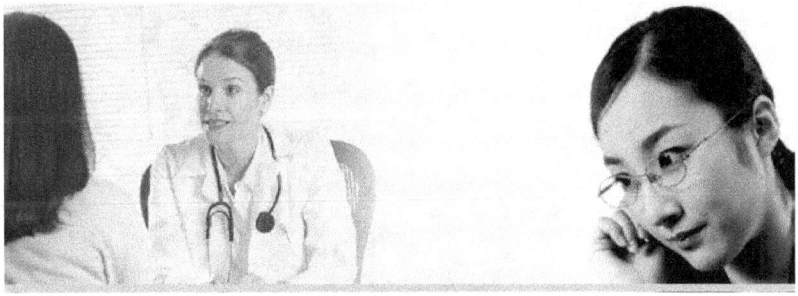

What is clinical research?

Clinical research refers to studies in which people participate as patients or volunteers. Different terms are used to describe clinical research, including clinical studies, clinical trials, studies, research, trials, and protocols. Clinical research may have a number of goals, such as developing new treatments or medications, identifying causes of illness, studying trends, or evaluating ways in which genetics may be related to an illness.

Strict rules for clinical studies have been put in place by NIH and the U.S. Food and Drug Administration (FDA). Some studies involve promising new treatments that may directly benefit participants. Others do not directly benefit participants, but may help scientists learn better ways to help people.

Confidentiality is an important part of clinical research and ensures that personal information is seen only by those authorized to have access. It also means that the personal identity and all medical information of clinical trial participants is known only to the individual patient and researchers. Results from a study will usually be presented only in terms of trends or overall findings and will not mention specific participants.

People sometimes think that participating in a study will require changes to their current treatment, but this is not always the case. Though some studies may require participants to try new medications or treatments, other studies use techniques such as brain scans, psychological tests, behavioral observation, or blood tests for genetic evaluation. Such studies may not require any change in treatment.

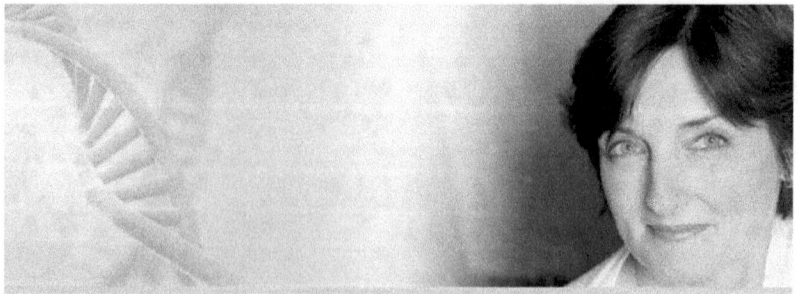

Why do people choose to participate in research?

People participate in research for several reasons. Some hope to get the most advanced treatment available for mental and behavioral illnesses. Others participate because they want to assist scientists in developing better ways to help people.

Research is our best hope for understanding and treating mental illnesses. Thanks to help from volunteers, medical researchers are learning more and more about the causes of mental and behavioral disorders, and are finding new ways to treat and prevent illnesses. Without this important relationship between research participants and those studying their illnesses, it would be much more difficult to improve health treatments.

Volunteers of all ethnic and cultural backgrounds are needed. By having a variety of volunteers participate, researchers can learn how different people react to medications and other treatments. For example, by studying the differences in men and women, researchers discovered that these groups have very different warning signs for a heart attack.

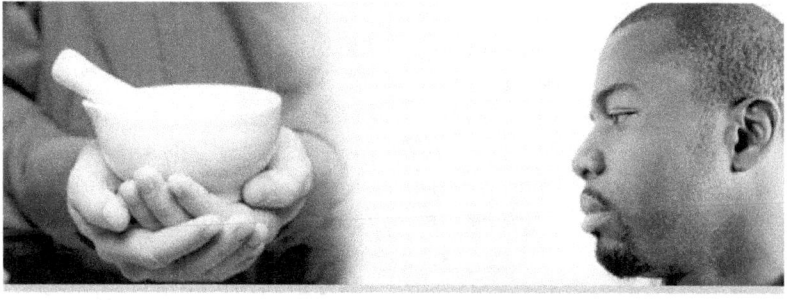

A comparison: participating in clinical research and seeing your doctor for treatment

Participating in clinical research is not the same as seeing your doctor. Here are some differences:

Participating in Clinical Research	Seeing Your Doctor
The researcher's goal is to learn about your illness.	Your doctor's goal is to treat your condition.
The researcher must use standardized procedures. You will probably be removed from the study if your illness worsens.	Your doctor will change your treatment as necessary.
You will be randomly assigned to a group taking a standard treatment or placebo, also known as an inactive pill (control group), or a group taking a new treatment (treatment group).	Your doctor will usually offer standard treatment for your illness.
The results from your participation may help researchers develop new treatments and may be published so that other researchers can learn.	Your treatment is designed to help you, not to help the doctor learn how to treat people with your illness.
In some cases, costs of the study may be covered, and you may receive additional compensation.	You will likely need to pay or use insurance for treatment.
With your permission, researchers may check in with your doctors to learn about your conditions and past treatments.	Your doctor usually won't share your information with researchers. (In some cases, he or she may ask permission to share information).

What are the different types of clinical research?

Different types of clinical research are used depending on what the researchers are studying. Below are descriptions of some different kinds of clinical research.

Treatment
Treatment research (also called "clinical trials") generally involves an intervention such as medication, psychotherapy, new devices, or new approaches to surgery or radiation therapy.

Prevention
Prevention research looks for better ways to prevent disorders from developing or returning. Different kinds of prevention research may study medicines, vitamins, vaccines, minerals, or lifestyle changes.

Diagnostic
This refers to the practice of looking for better ways to identify a particular disorder or condition.

Screening
Screening research aims to find the best ways to detect certain disorders or health conditions.

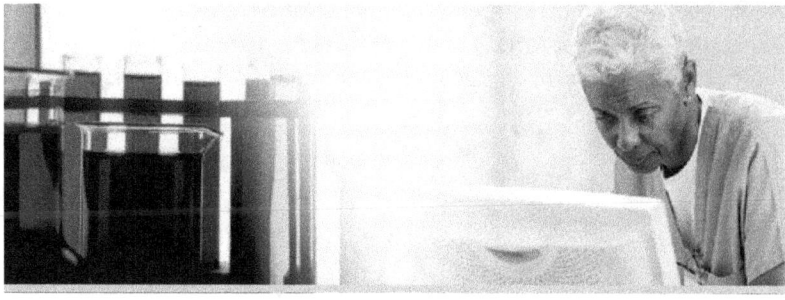

Quality of life
Also known as "supportive care," this research explores ways to improve comfort and the quality of life for individuals with a chronic illness.

Genetic studies
Genetic studies aim to improve the prediction of disorders by identifying and understanding how genes and illnesses may be related. Research in this area may explore ways in which a person's genes make him or her more or less likely to develop a disorder. This may lead to development of tailor-made treatments based on a patient's genetic make-up.

Epidemiological studies
Epidemiological studies seek to identify the patterns, causes, and control of disorders in groups of people.

An important note: some clinical research is "outpatient," meaning that participants do not stay overnight at the hospital. Some is "inpatient," meaning that participants will need to stay for at least one night in the hospital or research center. Be sure to ask the researchers what their study requires.

Phases of clinical trials: when clinical research is used to evaluate medications and devices

Clinical trials are a kind of clinical research designed to evaluate and test new interventions such as psychotherapy or medications. Clinical trials are often conducted in four phases. The trials at each phase have a different purpose and help scientists answer different questions.

Phase I trials
Researchers test an experimental drug or treatment in a small group of people for the first time. The researchers evaluate the treatment's safety, determine a safe dosage range, and identify side effects.

Phase II trials
The experimental drug or treatment is given to a larger group of people to see if it is effective and to further evaluate its safety.

Phase III trials
The experimental study drug or treatment is given to large groups of people. Researchers confirm its effectiveness, monitor side effects, compare it to commonly used treatments, and collect information that will allow the experimental drug or treatment to be used safely.

Phase IV trials
Post-marketing studies, which are conducted after a treatment is approved for use by the FDA, provide additional information including the treatment or drug's risks, benefits, and best use.

Examples of other kinds of clinical research

Many people believe that all clinical research involves testing of new medications or devices. This is not true, however. Some studies do not involve testing medications and a person's regular medications may not need to be changed. Healthy volunteers are also needed so that researchers can compare their results to results of people with the illness being studied. Some examples of other kinds of research include the following:

- A long-term study that involves psychological tests or brain scans
- A genetic study that involves blood tests but no changes in medication
- A study of family history that involves talking to family members to learn about people's medical needs and history.

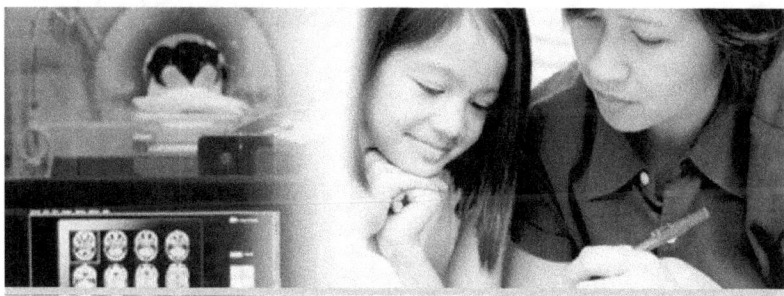

What are the risks and benefits of participating in research?

Clinical research can involve risk, but it is important to remember that routine medical care also involves risk. It is important that you weigh the risks and benefits of participating in research before enrolling. When thinking about risk, consider two important questions:

1. What is the chance that the study will cause me harm?

2. If there is a chance of harm, how much harm could I experience?

If you are interested in participating in a study, ask the researchers any questions that will help you decide whether to participate. Taking time to share your concerns will help you feel safe if you do decide to volunteer. (You can find sample questions at the end of this booklet.) It may be helpful to involve close family members, your doctors, or friends in this decision-making process.

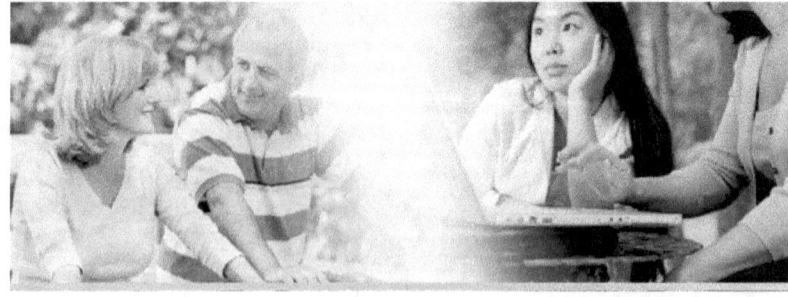

Risks

The nature of the risks depends on the kind of study. Often, clinical studies pose the risk of only minor discomfort that lasts for a short time. For example, in some mental health studies, participants take psychological tests; this is obviously a different kind of risk from undergoing surgery as part of a study. A participant in a study requiring surgery may risk greater complications. Risk can occur in many different ways, and it is important to speak with the research team to understand the risks in a particular study.

Keep in mind that all research sites are required to review their studies for any possible harm, and to share any potential risks with study volunteers. Possible risks include the following:

- The treatment involved may have health risks for you, such as unwanted side effects.
- The study may require more time and attention than standard treatment. You may need to visit the study site, take additional blood tests, stay in the hospital, or manage complex dosage requirements for medication.
- The treatment may not make you or other participants better.
- You may enroll in the study hoping to receive a new treatment, but you may be randomly assigned to receive a standard treatment or placebo (inactive pill).
- Whether a new treatment will work cannot be known ahead of time. There is always a chance that a new treatment may not work better than a standard treatment, may not work at all, or may be harmful.
- The treatment you receive may cause side effects that are serious enough to require medical attention.

Benefits

Benefits to participating in a study include:
- Treatment with experimental or study medications not widely available elsewhere.
- Care from a research team that includes doctors and other health care professionals who are familiar with the most advanced treatments available.
- Treatment that has been reviewed by many people, including other doctors and researchers.
- Research-related care or medicine at no cost.
- The opportunity to learn more about an illness and how to take care of it.
- The satisfaction of helping others by contributing to medical knowledge, or helping to identify possible new treatments.

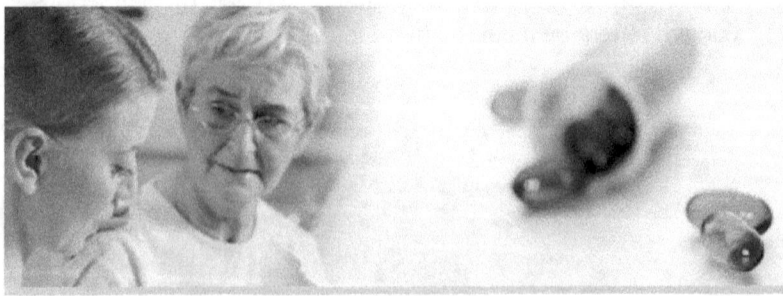

What rights do I have?

Deciding whether or not to participate

If you are eligible for a clinical study, you will be given information that will help you decide whether or not to take part. As a patient, you have the right to:
- Be told about important risks and benefits.
- Require confidentiality, or having maintained as private all personal medical information and personal identity.
- Know how the researchers plan to carry out the research, how long your participation will take, and where the study will take place.
- Know what is expected of you.
- Know any costs you or your insurers will be responsible for.
- Know if you will receive any financial compensation or reimbursement for expenses.
- Be informed about any medical or personal information that may be shared with other researchers directly involved in the clinical research.
- Talk openly with doctors and ask any questions.

Once you have decided to participate

After you join a clinical research study, you have the right to:
- Leave the study at any time. Participation is strictly voluntary. You can choose not to participate in any part of the research. However, you should not enroll if you do not plan to complete the study.
- Receive any new information that might affect your decision to be in the study.
- Continue to ask questions and get answers.
- Maintain your privacy. Neither your name nor any other identifying information will appear in any reports based on the study.
- Ask about your treatment assignment once the study is completed, if you participated in a study that randomly assigned you to a treatment group.

What are the possible financial costs?

In some clinical research studies, the medical facility conducting the research pays for your treatment and other expenses. In other trials, you may be responsible for costs. Be sure to ask about possible expenses.
- You or your health insurer may have to pay for some costs of your treatment that are considered part of standard care. This may include hospital stays, laboratory and other tests, and medical procedures.
- If you have health insurance, find out exactly what it will cover. If you don't have health insurance, or if your insurance company will not cover your costs, talk to the researchers or their staff about other options for covering the cost of your care.
- You also may need to pay for travel between your home and the clinic.

Who can participate in clinical research?

Each clinical research study has different requirements that determine whether a person can participate. These requirements are called "inclusion" and "exclusion" criteria. The criteria are used to help researchers answer the study questions and to ensure the safety of all volunteers.

Depending on what the study is testing, inclusion and exclusion criteria may include a person's:
- Illness
- Health history
- Past or current treatment
- Age or sex
- Address (A person living too far from where the study takes place may not be eligible to participate).

What is randomization?

In clinical research studies that seek to test the effectiveness of a new intervention (for example: a new medication or a new psychotherapy technique), participants will usually be evenly placed in different study groups. Participants do not know to which group they have been assigned. One group receives the experimental intervention; the other receives standard or no treatment. This process, called randomization, allows researchers to compare results between the two groups. It is important to note that many studies—such as those involving brain imaging or genetics—may not require randomization.

People who take part in studies requiring randomization are generally placed in a group based on chance, not choice. Some participants are placed in the "experimental" group, and the others are placed in the "control" group. The control group will receive standard treatment, a placebo, or other intervention based on the design of the study.

To understand how this works, imagine that 100 people decide to participate in a study that compares a new treatment to a standard treatment. Each participant is randomly assigned to either the treatment group or the control group. To do this, researchers use a "coin toss" or similar method. Half of the people are assigned to the treatment group and half are assigned to the control group. The researchers then compare the results of the two groups to see which treatment works better. They also try to figure out why it works better. The picture below helps explain how randomization works.

Clinical Research Participants (100 people)

Random placement into each group (like a coin toss)

Experimental Group (50 people)
Receive new medication or therapy

Control Group (50 people)
Receive a standard treatment with known effects

What is informed consent?

Before you take part in a study, it is important to fully understand it and to understand what participation may be like. Researchers will help by providing an "informed consent" statement. This is a document that has detailed information about the study, including its length, the number of visits required, and the medical procedures and medications in which you will take part. The document also provides expected outcomes, potential benefits, possible risks, any available treatment alternatives, expenses, terms of confidentiality, and contact information for people you can call if you have questions or concerns. When needed, a translator may be provided.

Researchers will review the informed consent statement with you and answer your questions. If you decide to participate after reviewing the statement, getting all the information you need, and talking with staff and your family, you will need to sign the informed consent statement. Your signature indicates that you understand the study and agree to participate voluntarily. You may still leave a study at any time and for any reason even after signing the informed consent document.

Sometimes, a potential participant may not be able to give informed consent because of memory problems or mental confusion. Someone else, usually a family member with a durable power of attorney, can give consent for that participant. That caregiver must be confident there is small risk to the participant, and that he or she would have agreed to consent if able to do so.

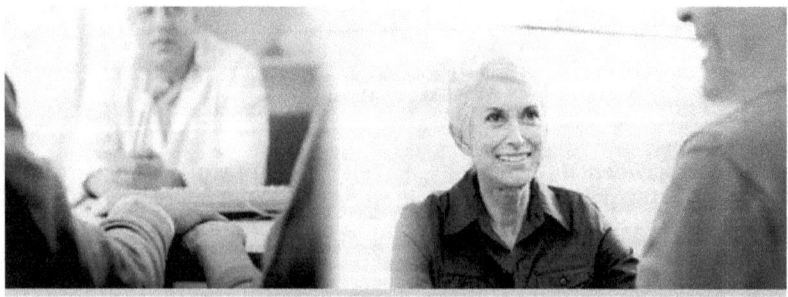

What else should I consider?

You should consider whether you want to empower someone you trust to make health decisions for you if you become sick. This is very important if you choose to participate in a study that changes your regular medication routine, and you and the researchers are unsure about how your body will react. For example, if your thinking becomes impaired, you might make a decision that you would not make if you were thinking clearly. In this case, you may want someone you trust to make a decision for you.

You are not always required to name someone else to make decisions if you become impaired. If you wish to do so, however, speak to the researcher to make sure he or she understands what you want; you may also want to ask what kind of paperwork is required to ensure that your representative will be contacted.

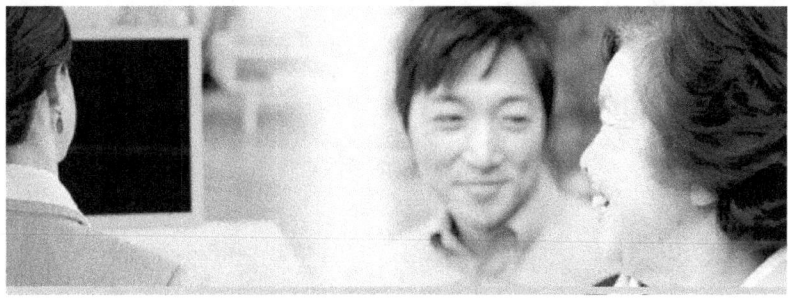

How do researchers make sure that participants are safe?

It's a good idea to ask questions and gather information before you make a decision about participating in research. It's also important to remember that strict rules protect participants in research studies. Researchers take these rules very seriously because they care about participants' health. Additionally, researchers must follow the rules if they want to be allowed to do more research.

Below is information about how study participants are kept safe.

Federal agencies
- Protect the rights and well-being of clinical research participants. Federal agencies including the FDA and NIH oversee much of the medical research in the United States.

Informed consent
- Informed consent is the process of learning about a clinical research study before you decide if you want to participate. For more information about informed consent, see the "What is informed consent?" section in this guide.

Institutional review boards (IRBs)
- IRBs oversee the research centers where clinical studies are conducted. IRBs review and approve study protocols (plans) for scientific merit, participant safety, and ethical considerations. Participants who have questions may contact the IRBs at the research center they are considering. IRB members usually include scientific experts as well as community members.

Leaving the trial
- Participants who wish to leave the trial because they feel unsafe may do so without penalty.

Peer review
- Federal agencies may review individuals and institutions conducting research.

Primary health care
- If you participate in a study, talk with your regular doctor to be sure that medications you normally take are safe to use with any medications you may take for the study. Sometimes the researcher will ask for permission to speak with your regular doctors to make sure you get the best treatment.

Protocol
- A protocol is a plan that details what researchers will do during a study. Every study must have a protocol. The protocol includes information on how researchers will work to keep participants safe.

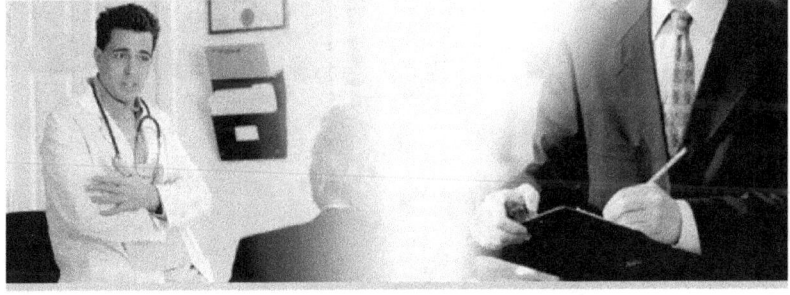

What kinds of results will come from the research?

- Researchers will sum up what they learned from the study.
  - Researchers will never identify you individually. They usually discuss trends and sometimes provide examples or stories, if they can do so without identifying participants.
- If you would like to know what the researcher learns from the study, ask how and when you can expect to find out about the results.
  - The researcher may suggest that you contact the study's office at a certain time, that you provide your contact information so study results can be mailed or e-mailed to you, or that you check online.
- A frustrating thing about research is that it can take a long time to complete. Sometimes, years may pass between the time you were involved in the study and the time when results become available.
  - The researchers may need to work with many more participants after you, and then analyze all the results.
  - Check in with the researcher if you do not hear about results at the expected time.

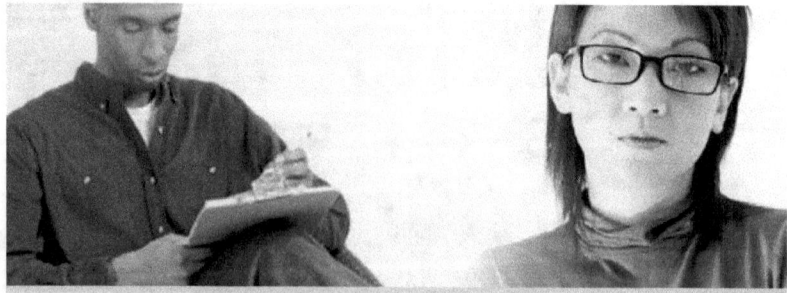

How can I enroll in clinical research?

As a starting point for information on NIMH research studies, visit the NIMH Web site at **http://www.nimh.nih.gov/health/trials/index.shtml**. NIH also maintains a database that includes information on clinical trials. The Web site address is **http://clinicaltrials.gov**. This Web site provides information on Federally funded and other clinical trials.

On **clinicaltrials.gov**, a contact person and phone number or e-mail address is usually listed with each study description. Information about clinical studies is also sometimes advertised in local newspapers, magazines, or on radio and television.

For a clinical study that you may have heard about or seen advertised, you can contact the clinical trial or study coordinator. You can find this information in the description. Your health care provider may also want to talk to this person about your health conditions. The first step after finding out about a study is to set up a screening appointment. During this appointment, researchers will ask you questions and may test you to see if you meet the needs of the study.

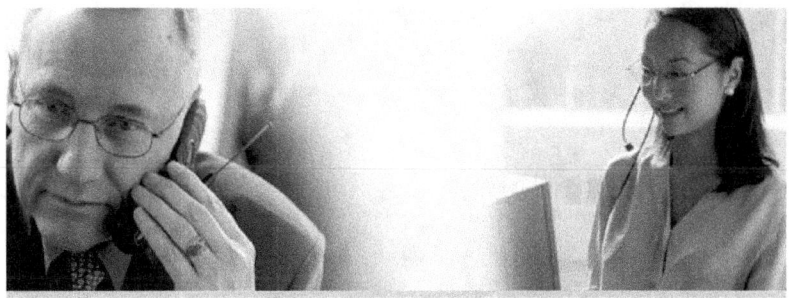

What kinds of questions should I ask the researcher?

As a participant, you are a partner in the study. It is important that you know what is likely to happen during the study and the purpose of the research.

One good way to find out about whether you want to participate is to ask the researcher questions. Below are some ideas about what to ask. Feel free to add your own questions.

- Why do you want me in your study?
- What is the research about? How will this research help doctors treat or understand my disorder?
- How might this study help me, my relatives, or other people with my disorder?
- Will taking part in this study affect my daily life?
- What are the standard treatments for my illness or condition?
- What is likely to happen to me without a new treatment?
- Are there risks for me if I participate? If so, what are they?
- Will this study involve any change in my medications?

Remember to ask again if you would like further explanation or if you did not understand the answer you received. You are entitled to understand! If you forget to ask a question or forget the answers to the questions, ask again. It is part of the researcher's job to help you understand.

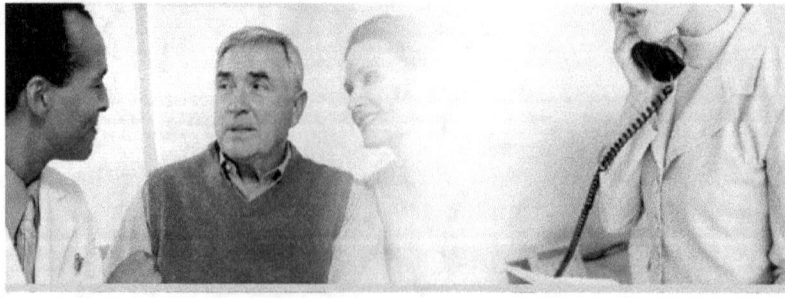

Glossary

Essential terms for understanding mental health clinical research

Comparison–To learn more, researchers compare results from patients in the experimental groups with results from patients in the control groups.

Confidentiality regarding participants–This refers to the practice of maintaining as private all information related to clinical trial participants, including their personal identity and all personal medical information. Results from the study will usually be presented in terms of trends or overall findings and will not mention any specific participants.

Control group–The group of participants that receives standard treatment or a placebo. The control group may also be made up of healthy volunteers. Researchers compare results from the control group with results from the experimental group to find and learn from any differences.

Double-blind research design–A study in which neither the participant nor the researcher knows whether the participant is in the treatment or control group.

Durable power of attorney–The authority to act for another person in specified or all legal or financial matters.

Double-blind, randomized, controlled clinical trial–This is a clinical trial in which the researchers evenly divide study participants into a group receiving the experimental intervention and a group receiving standard or no treatment. Neither group knows how it has been assigned. This practice reduces the chance for a "placebo effect," in which a treatment with no active ingredient produces results expected from a treatment with an active ingredient.

Experiment–A study done to answer a question. Other words to describe an experiment are "research," "study," and "protocol."

Experimental group–The group of participants in a study that receive the experimental or study intervention (such as medication or psychotherapy).

Food and Drug Administration (FDA)–The FDA is the Federal agency responsible for ensuring that foods are safe, wholesome and sanitary; human and veterinary drugs, biological products, and medical devices are safe and effective; cosmetics are safe; and electronic products that emit radiation are safe. Some of the agency's specific responsibilities include regulating medications and devices.

Healthy volunteer–In a clinical study, a person who does not have the disorder or disease being studied. Results from healthy controls are compared to results from the group being studied.

Inclusion/exclusion criteria–Inclusion criteria are the factors that allow someone to participate in a clinical trial. Exclusion criteria are the factors that prevent someone from participating in the trial. These factors may include a person's illness, health history, past treatment, age, sex, or where he or she lives.

Informed consent–When a participant provides informed consent, it means that he or she has learned the key facts about a research study and agrees to take part in it. For more detailed information, see the "What is informed consent?" section in this guide.

Inpatient–A person who is hospitalized for at least one night to receive treatment or participate in a study.

National Institutes of Health (NIH)–Part of the U.S. Department of Health and Human Services, NIH is the primary Federal agency for conducting and supporting medical research. NIH scientists investigate ways to prevent disease as well as the causes, treatments, and even cures for common and rare diseases. Composed of 27 Institutes and Centers, NIH provides leadership and financial support to researchers in every state and throughout the world.

Outpatient–A person who receives treatment or participates in a study but is not hospitalized overnight.

Placebo–An inactive pill. This is sometimes called a "sugar pill." In some studies, participants may be assigned to take a placebo rather than the study medication. Ask the researcher if this is a possibility for the study that interests you.

Placebo effect–Sometimes people taking a study medication receive benefits that are not from the chemicals in the medicine. This is called a "placebo effect." For example, if a participant feels hopeful about a treatment, he or she may be more likely to notice positive changes than negatives ones. A researcher's hope may also sway a participant's response. Double-blind research design helps minimize the placebo effect.

Post-marketing studies–Studies done after a treatment, medication or device is approved for use by the FDA. These studies gather additional information about a product's safety, effectiveness, or best use.

Protocol–A study done to answer a question. Other words to describe a protocol are "research," "study," and "experiment." "Protocol" also refers to the plan that details what researchers will do during the study.

Randomization/random assignment–This is the process in which researchers evenly assign study participants into a group receiving the experimental treatment being studied, and others into a group receiving standard or no treatment. Participants are assigned to a group based on chance, not choice. You have the same chance to be placed in any of the test groups.

Research–A study done to answer a question. Scientists do research when they're not sure what will work best to help people with an illness. Other words to describe clinical research are "clinical trial," "protocol," "study," and "experiment."

Sponsors–Clinical trials are sponsored or funded by various organizations or individuals, including physicians, foundations, medical institutions, voluntary groups, and pharmaceutical companies, as well as Federal agencies such as NIH, FDA, the Department of Defense, and the Department of Veterans Affairs.

Standard treatment–The treatment that medical professionals consider at the time of the study to be the most prevalent and best available treatment.

Standardized procedures–These are study rules that researchers must follow exactly for every participant, regardless of what each participant is used to. For example, if you normally take a medicine by injection but the experiment is testing the same medicine in pill form, the researcher must prescribe pills to you. The researcher cannot use a different method for you.

Study–Conducted by a principal investigator who is often a doctor. Members of the research team regularly monitor the participant's health to determine the study's safety and effectiveness. Other words to describe a study are "clinical trial," "protocol," "experiment," and "research."

Single-blind research design–A study in which one party, either the investigator or participant, is unaware of what medication or intervention the participant is taking; also called single-masked study.

References

1. NIH Clinical Center: **http://clinicalresearch.nih.gov**
2. ClinicalTrials.gov: Glossary of Clinical Trials Terms
   http://clinicaltrials.gov/ct2/info/glossary
3. National Cancer Institute: **http://www.cancer.gov/dictionary**

For more information on clinical research and clinical trials

- Visit the National Library of Medicine's MedlinePlus
  http://medlineplus.gov
  En Español **http://medlineplus.gov/spanish**
- Information on mental health clinical trials
  http://www.nimh.nih.gov/health/trials/index.shtml
- National Library of Medicine Clinical Trials Database
  http://www.clinicaltrials.gov

Information from NIMH is available in multiple formats. You can browse online, download documents in PDF, and order paper brochures through the mail. If you would like to have NIMH publications, you can order them online at: **http://www.nimh.nih.gov**.

For the most up-to-date information on this topic, please check the NIMH Web site at: **http://www.nimh.nih.gov**.

If you do not have Internet access and wish to have information that supplements this publication, please contact the NIMH Information Resource Center at the following numbers:

National Institute of Mental Health
Science Writing, Press & Dissemination Branch
6001 Executive Boulevard
Room 8184, MSC 9663
Bethesda, MD 20892-9663
Phone: 301-443-4513 or
1-866-615–NIMH (6464) toll-free
TTY: 301-443-8431 or
1-866-415-8051 toll-free
FAX: 301-443-4279
E-mail: **nimhinfo@nih.gov**
Web site: **http://www.nimh.nih.gov**

Reprints:

This publication is in the public domain and may be reproduced or copied without permission from NIMH. We encourage you to reproduce it and use it in your efforts to improve public health. Citation of the National Institute of Mental Health as a source is appreciated. However, using government materials inappropriately can raise legal or ethical concerns, so we ask you to use these guidelines:

- NIMH does not endorse or recommend any commercial products, processes, or services, and our publications may not be used for advertising or endorsement purposes.
- NIMH does not provide specific medical advice or treatment recommendations or referrals; our materials may not be used in a manner that has the appearance of such information.
- NIMH requests that non-Federal organizations not alter our publications in ways that will jeopardize the integrity and "brand" when using the publication.
- Addition of non-Federal Government logos and Web site links may not have the appearance of NIMH endorsement of any specific commercial products or services or medical treatments or services.

If you have questions regarding these guidelines and use of NIMH publications, please contact the NIMH Information Resource Center at 1–866–615–6464 or e-mail at nimhinfo@nih.gov.

The photos in this publication are of models and are used for illustrative purposes only.